Blood Pressure
BY EMILY HOSKINS

Blood Pressure Solution - Lower Your Blood Pressure Using Natural Remedies

Second Edition

Copyright

Blood Pressure: Blood Pressure Solution - Lower Your Blood Pressure Using Natural Remedies

Second Edition – June 2015

Emily Hoskins

Disclaimer Notice

Please note the information contained within this document is for educational and entertainment purposes only. Every attempt has been made to provide accurate, up to date and reliable complete information. No warranties of any kind are expressed or implied. Readers acknowledge that the author is not engaging in the rendering of legal, financial, medical or professional advice.

By reading this document, the reader agrees that under no circumstances are we responsible for any losses, direct or indirect, which are incurred as a result of the use of information contained within this document, including, but not limited to, —errors, omissions, or inaccuracies.

Table of Contents

Introduction

High blood pressure is one of the most widespread conditions in the world. In the USA alone, one in three adults suffer with it and over 50% of those do not have the condition under control. High blood pressure, otherwise known as hypertension is a silent killer. There may not be any signs or symptoms of high blood pressure until it becomes severe. However, that doesn't mean that the damage is not already being done inside your body.

There is a good chance that you are downloading this eBook either because you have just had your blood pressure tested and it's a little high or you've been suffering with hypertension for some time now but really don't want to be popping pills for the rest of your life. So what can you do?

Even if you don't have high blood pressure now, you should always make sure you have it checked regularly so that any changes can be picked up on early enough. You can buy a blood pressure machine to use at home if you like. In terms of treatment, there are, outside of medication, three natural ways to treat hypertension – diet, exercise and a reduction in stress. These three are what we are going to focus on in this eBook.

Chapter 1: What is High Blood Pressure?

High blood pressure, or hypertension, is when there is too much blood pressure on blood vessel walls. Very often, someone who has high blood pressure will not present with any symptoms until the condition is severe. When the heart pumps, it pushes blood through your arteries and throughout your body. Pressure may be caused by blood pressing on the artery walls and, each beat of the heart pushes even more blood through, causing that pressure to go up. Between heartbeats, the pressure should lower.

Most of us have had our blood pressure taken at some time or another; the doctor will place a cuff around the arm and inflate it using warm air. He or she then listens to the flow of your blood using a stethoscope. The numbers they come up with for your blood pressure reading are based on your heartbeat – systolic pressure – and the resting period between each beat – diastolic pressure. A normal blood pressure reading is less than 120 mm HG systolic and 80 mm HG diastolic, usually written as 120/80. Any reading higher than 140/90 could be an indication of high blood pressure.

- Pre-hypertension: 10-139, over 30-89

- Stage 1 hypertension: 140-159, over 90-99

- Stage 2 hypertension: 160 and above, over 100 and above

- Hypertension among people of 60 years: 150 and above, over 90 and above

Types of high blood pressure

- Essential or primary hypertension/ high blood pressure

This is a kind of high blood pressure that will develop gradually over a number of years.

- Secondary hypertension/ high blood pressure

This type of high blood pressure is caused by an underlying factor and tends to show up suddenly. It can be caused by a number of health complications such as

- Thyroid problems

- Kidney problems

- Adrenal gland tumors

- Certain congenital blood vessel

- Some medications, for example birth control pills, some prescription drugs, decongestants, cold remedies, and over-the-counter pain relievers

- Obstructive sleep apnea

- Illegal drugs, such as cocaine and amphetamines

- Alcohol abuse or chronic alcohol use

What Causes It?

In most cases the cause is not known and this is called primary or essential hypertension. When the cause of the high blood pressure is known, it is called secondary hypertension and some of the causes include blood vessel or kidney abnormalities that can be corrected. Although we don't always know the root cause of the hypertension, we do know that there are certain factors that will exacerbate it:

- **Smoking** – Nicotine makes the blood vessels shrink, or constrict, making the force of the blood pressure much higher

- **Obesity** – carrying extra weight puts strain on the heart and, while exercise can help you to lose weight, it has also been shown to bring blood pressure down, even in those who are not overweight

- **Stress** – not a cause of high blood pressure, stress can certainly trigger off bad habits that will affect blood pressure, like over eating, drinking and smoking

- **Salt** – Sodium makes your body hold on to fluid which, in turn, increases blood pressure

- **Alcohol** – Drinking more than the recommended allowance can affect blood pressure for some people.

- **Race** – High blood pressure is more prevalent among blacks and they tend to develop it at an earlier ages compared to whites. They are also highly prone to other health complications such as kidney failure, stroke and heart attack.

- **Living a physically inactive life** – Going to the gym to work out is not about showing off but making sure that your body is not inactive. People who lead such an active life are not prone to getting high blood pressure while their inactive counterparts are. This is because the higher one's heart rate is, the harder the heart works at every contraction hence a stronger force exerted on one's arteries. An inactive life also increases chances of obesity.

- **Age** – One's likelihood to get high blood pressure increases with increase in age. Among men, the chances get higher in their middle age or 45 years while among women, it is after 65 years.

- **Family history** – One may also get high blood pressure simply because it runs in the family.

- **Insufficient potassium in one's diet** – Potassium is important in one's diet for it helps balance the amount of sodium one's cells have. Little potassium in the diet or failure to retain enough potassium means an accumulation of sodium in one's blood which brings on high blood pressure

- **Insufficient vitamin D in one's diet** – It is not certain that little amounts of vitamin D in one's diet causes high blood pressure. However, its insufficiency affects an enzyme that is produced by our kidneys which affects one's blood pressure.

- **Chronic health complications** – There are some chronic health conditions that are likely to increase one's chances of developing high blood pressure. These include, sleep apnea, kidney disease.

- **Pregnancy** – It is not to say that every pregnant woman develops high blood pressure, however, there are some that develop it. All this is due to the many changes that the body undergoes when one becomes pregnant. Pregnant women need to attend all their doctor's visits or antenatal classes for it is during these visits that such issues will be seen. High blood pressure in this instance is very dangerous and should not be ignored at all.

While hypertension is prevalent among older people, children are also becoming prone to it. Among children, high blood pressure is brought on by health complications pertaining to the heart or kidneys. In addition to that, a number of children have poor lifestyle habits like obesity, inactive lives, unhealthy diets that bring on high blood pressure.

How Hypertension Affects Health

As your heart pumps blood, it goes through the arteries and into blood vessels, which gradually become smaller and more delicate. The smallest vessels are called capillaries and these are responsible for supplying oxygen to your body. If the pressure within this life-support system increases, your heart has to work harder. This can lead to damage to the arteries and, as a result, because they are not receiving sufficient oxygen, the following organs will also be affected:

- **Brain** - high blood pressure can be responsible for vessels within the brain rupturing and these ruptures or blood clots can cause a stroke

- **Eyes** – High blood pressure can also cause vessels in the eye to rupture, causing problems with vision and possibly blindness

- **Kidneys** – If the blood vessels constrict too much your kidneys can lose the ability to effectively filter waste products out of the blood and this can result in kidney failure which may need dialysis or transplant to cure

- **Heart** – the heart needs oxygenated blood to survive. If it doesn't get sufficient amounts, or the flow of blood to the heart is blocked, the result could be angina or heart attack. And, as your heat has to work harder to pump the blood around, it could result in congestive heart failure.

High blood pressure itself is not a disease but it can quickly cause these other problems in your body. These problems include:

- **Aneurysm** – When blood pressure increases, it causes one's blood vessels to weaken and bulge which leads to aneurysm. One's life gets even more threatened should the aneurysm rupture.

- **Heart failure** – With increased blood pressure, pumping blood causes the heart muscle to become thick. This thickened muscle will have difficulty in pumping blood that is sufficient enough as to meet the needs of the whole body. This in turn leads to heart failure.

- **Metabolic syndrome** – This is a collection of disorders in one's metabolism. These disorders include high triglycerides, high insulin levels, increased waist circumference, low high-density lipoprotein (HDL), high blood pressure, and cholesterol. High blood pressure usually causes metabolic syndrome components, which make one susceptible to stroke, diabetes.

- **Problems with understanding and/or memory Trouble** – When high blood pressure is on the rise, one's ability to learn, think or remember is affected. People with high blood pressure usually have trouble with understanding and memory.

And, although it isn't a disease, it does have an underlying cause – a cause that can normally be fixed with the following lifestyle changes. We're going to start by looking at your diet.

Chapter 2: How to Lower Your Blood Pressure with Diet

One of the easiest ways to bring your blood pressure down is through diet. Many people who have hypertension are overweight and are often told by their doctors that they must lose weight to bring their blood pressure down. The Cochrane Collaboration carried out a number of tests to see if there is any scientific evidence that this is true, using suitable studies that showed whether there was any correlation between diet and blood pressure.

They look at eight different studies, with a collective number of 2100 participants, showing the effect of different diets on blood pressure. Most of the studies lasted for a period of 12 months and, on average, the participants lost around 4 kg, or 9 lbs., resulting in a lowering of the blood pressure. On average, the systolic value dropped by 4.5 mm HG and the diastolic value by 3 mm HG.

They also looked at four studies that tested the drug Orlistat in conjunction with diet and the results showed that the participants in these studies lost an average of 4 kg over a period between 6 and 48 months. The average systolic value dropped by 2.5 mm HG and the diastolic by 2 mm HG. It must be said though that Orlistat does cause a number of side effects with the most common one being digestion problems.

Cut the Salt

Reducing the amount of salt you eat is one of the quickest ways to bring your blood pressure down. Salt has been proven to raise blood pressure and the more you eat, the higher your pressure goes. It does this because it makes you retain water. The more salt you eat, the more water you retain and this can push your blood pressure higher. On top of that, if you are on medication for blood pressure, such as diuretics, the salt will counteract the effectiveness of them.

To cut down on your salt intake, the best thing to do is eat foods that are low-sodium and not add extra, either during cooking or at the table. Read the labels on the food you buy to see how much salt is in it:

- 0.3 g or less to 100 g of food – low salt, you can at plenty of this type

- 0.3 – 1.5 g to 100 g of food – medium salt, eat occasionally and in small amounts

- 1.5 g or more per 100 g of food – high salt, to be avoided completely

If you can't see how much salt is in a food item on the label, take a look at the list of ingredients – the nearer the top of the ingredients list it appears, the more slat is in it.

How to Eat less Salt and Lower Your Blood Pressure

- Do not add salt to food you are preparing or cooking – that includes stock cubes, curry powder, soy sauce, etc.

- Use herbs and spices instead of salt for flavorings, along with seasonings like lemon juice, lime juice, chili or ginger

- If you can't eat food with salty flavor, try a low-sodium substitute

- Check the labels on table sauces, like pickles, mustard or ketchup – they contain high levels of salt so should be avoided if possible

- Bread contains salt as do many breakfast cereals – check the labels before you buy

- Smoked fish and smoked meat contain a high level of salt, avoid them if you can

- If you go to a restaurant to eat, ask the chef to use less salt in your meal – they may not be able to do it but it is always worth asking

- Look for recipes that use less salt

You should eat no more than 6 g of salt per day so just look for the lowest salt options on your groceries.

What Your Diet Should Consist of:

Grains – 6-8 servings per day

Grains can be found in bread, pasta, cereal and rice. One serving would be 1 slice of whole grain bread or ½ cup of cooked rice, pasta or cereal. Try to go for whole grain as they contain more nutrients and fiber. For example, use whole-wheat pasta, brown rice and whole grain bread instead of white.

Vegetables – 4-5 servings per day

Lots of vegetables are full of fiber and vitamins, as well as minerals like magnesium and potassium. One serving would be 1 cup of raw leafy green vegetable, like spinach or kale, or ½ cup of chopped up vegetables like tomatoes, sweet potatoes, greens, or carrots, either raw or cooked. Use either fresh or frozen vegetables but do check the salt levels on frozen or canned.

Fruit – 4-5 servings per day

Many fruits are full of fiber, magnesium and potassium and require little to no preparation to become a staple part of your diet. Most are low in fat, with the exception of avocado and coconut and a serving would be one medium piece of fruit or ½ cup of fresh, canned or frozen fruit. You can also count 4 oz. of fruit juice as one serving. Try not to peel your fruit if it does not need it. Things like apple and pear skins contain fiber and nutrients. If you do choose juice or canned fruit, make sure it is sugar free. And, if you are on any medications, check with your doctor because citrus fruits can have a negative effect on certain ones.

Dairy – 2-3 servings per day

Dairy foods like cheese, milk and yoghurt are a big source of calcium, protein and vitamin D but you should be looking for low fat or fat free products, to reduce your intake of saturated fats. One serving would be 1 cup of 1% or skim milk, 1 ½ oz. cheese or 1 cup of yoghurt. Add fruit to yoghurt for the perfect sweet treat.

Poultry, fish or meat – 6 or fewer servings per day

Meat contains vitamin B, zinc, iron and protein but you should always choose a lean version. Don't eat too much meat because it contains fat and cholesterol – cut your meat portion back, and top up with vegetables instead. One serving would be 1 oz. of poultry, cooked with the skin off, seafood or lean meat or an egg.

Nuts, Legumes and Seeds – 4-5 servings per week

Kidney beans, sunflower seeds, almonds, lentils, peas and other similar foods are full of protein, potassium and magnesium, as well as phytochemicals and fiber, which can protect against certain cancers and heart disease. Because these foods are so high in calories, you should eat no more than 4-5 servings per week and a serving would be 1-½ oz. nuts, ½ cup cooked beans or peas or 2 tablespoons of seeds.

Fats and oils – 2-3 servings per day

Fat is an essential part of your diet because it helps your body to absorb the vitamins in your food and it helps to build up the immune system. Too much can cause heart disease, obesity and diabetes. Less than 27% of your total daily calories should come from fat, preferably monounsaturated fats. One serving is 1 tablespoon of mayonnaise, 1 teaspoon of soft margarine or 2 tablespoons of salad dressing. Definitely avoid anything that has Trans fats in it, generally found in processed foods.

Sweets – 5 or less per week

You do not have to throw out all your sweet stuff; just take it easy, one serving would be 1 tablespoon of sugar jam or jelly, 8 oz. lemonade or ½ cup of sorbet. Choose sweets that are low in fat and sugar. While artificial sweeteners may be a good substitute for sugar, use them as sensibly as you would sugar.

Alcohol and Caffeine

Too much alcohol will raise your blood pressure and you should stick to no more than 2 units per day if you are a man or 1 if you are a woman. While we know that caffeine will raise blood pressure, it isn't clear how much is a bad thing. So, the advice is to be sensible and limit how much you drink and, if you think that it is having a bad effect on your blood pressure, cut down or switch to decaffeinate. However, when you are eliminating caffeine from your diet, you need to do gradually over a period of time to avoid getting withdrawal symptoms such as headaches.

Consume Foods Rich in Omega 3 And 6 Fats

Foods rich in Omega 3 fats are flaxseed oil, fish, walnut oil but fish has the highest amount of these 3. Foods rich in Omega 6 fats are safflower, corn, sunflower oil, soy and canola. Omega 3 fats help in re-sensitizing insulin receptors for one suffering from insulin resistance.

These 2 fats are needed in particular quantities, a ratio 6:3 but most people tend to consume more of the foods containing Omega 6 fats. Consuming a lot of Omega 6 fat rich foods is not healthy for our bodies. The other problem that is arising is that most fresh fish today is loaded with high levels of mercury, which is harmful to our bodies. Therefore you need to find a safe source of fish to avoid consuming mercury. If that option seems difficult, high quality krill oil would be great for it has been found to have lots of Omega 3, even higher than that found in fish oil.

Eat Fermented Foods

When naturally fermented foods such as kefir, yogurt, natto, sauerkraut and other fermented vegetables are consumed, they help in optimizing one's gut flora. This is because the difference between one's gut flora from another person has been seen to have a huge effect on whether one will develop heart complications or not. Healthy gut flora means that one is not prone to heart complications and many other chronic health issues.

Fermented foods are also a great source of vitamin K2, which helps in alleviating arterial plaque buildup and heart complications.

To Get the Best Out Of Your Diet

Making sudden changes to your diet won't make you feel very good to start with and you are less likely to stick with it. Instead, change things gradually. If you already eat two servings of vegetables a day, add another one in and reduce your meat consumption. Add in fruits, vegetables and whole grains gradually to give your body chance to get used to it – too much at once can make you feel bloated and give you diarrhea.

Adding physical activity to your diet will give you the best results but we will talk more about that in the next chapter. Eating a healthy diet isn't an all-or nothing – even making some changes to your diet will help and you should slowly make the changes – swap out that chocolate bar for an apple or that cheesy pastry for a portion of vegetables or a salad. Keep your diet interesting to ensure you stick to it – boredom is the biggest reason for people failing their diets.

Chapter 3: How to Lower Your High Blood Pressure with Herbs and Supplements

There are a number of ways to lower your hypertension such as medication, change of lifestyle and the like. However, if you would like to use herbal and traditional treatments, there are many options available to you, most of which are in your back yard garden.

When you make up your mind to make use of herbs or their supplements, it will be wise to consult your doctor before using them. This is because while some herbs and supplements are okay from all angles, some could bring hazardous side effects when using in large quantities while others could interfere with other medications already in use. Here are some herbs and supplements that can be used to help lower you blood pressure naturally:

Cardamom

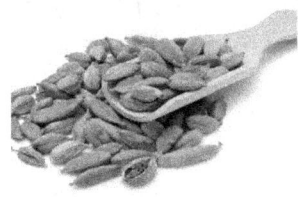 This seasoning herb has its origins in India and is usually used in South Asian foods. A study has revealed that persons who consume cardamom powder on a daily basis will definitely have low blood pressure. Cardamom seeds and powder can also be used in soups, spice rubs and baking for great flavor and great health benefits.

Cinnamon

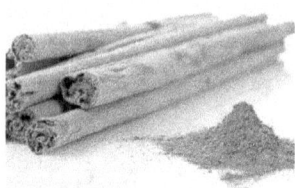

This herb is tasty and used a lot in seasoning. It is simple to include in your diet and it will help lower your blood pressure a bit. Cinnamon is said to help diabetic people lower their blood pressure. Sprinkle a little cinnamon into your breakfast cereal, coffee, tea and oatmeal. It can also be used to enhance the flavor of stews, fries and curries for a splendid meal.

Celery seed

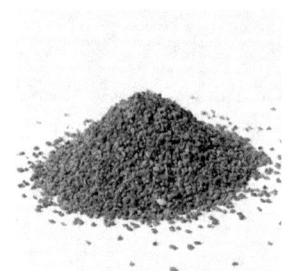

This herb is used to add flavor to casseroles, soups, stews and many more savory dishes. It has been used for a number of years by Chinese as a treatment for hypertension and studies indicate its effectiveness. The seeds can also be used to lower high blood pressure; however making juice out of the whole plant would also be great. Celery is effective when dealing with high blood pressure because it is a diuretic.

Basil

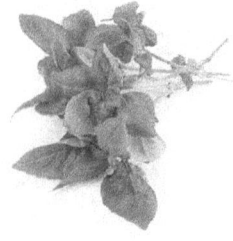

This herb is delicious and used a lot when cooking. It is also said to help lower blood pressure, however it does this for just a short period of time. You could also add fresh basil into your diet and no harm will be done. Grow this in your back yard if you do not have it already and add its fresh leaves to your casseroles, soups, pastas and salads.

Garlic

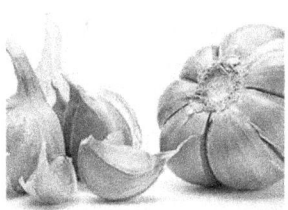

Not many people love garlic because it gives off a pungent smell but this seasoning clove does more than flavor food while ruining your breath. Garlic helps in lowering high blood pressure as it makes blood vessel relax and dilate. This then causes blood to flow a whole lot more freely and high blood pressure is reduced. Fresh garlic can be added to a series of recipes however if you find the flavor too strong, roast it first. One could also eat it raw or get it in form of supplements.

Hawthorn

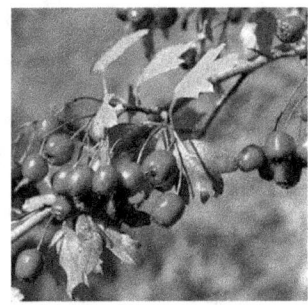

This herbal remedy has been in use mainly among Chinese and it has been in use for thousands of years. Hawthorn extractions seem to have a lot of benefits for cardiovascular health such as reducing high blood pressure, preventing formation of clots, increasing circulation of blood. You can choose to take hawthorn as a liquid extract, tea or pill.

Cat's claw

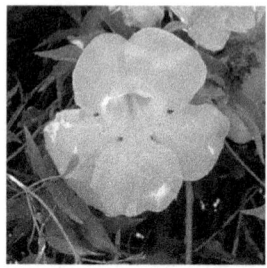 This herb is used as herbal medicine in traditional Chinese medicine as a treatment for neurological health complications as well as hypertension. Research shows that cat's claw works well to lower high blood pressure by acting on the calcium channels within one's cells. Cat's claw is available as a supplement in several health stores.

French Lavender

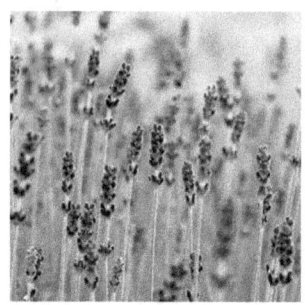 French lavender has got a perfume like scent and it is beautiful hence used for aesthetic purposes. Its oil is used as a perfume ingredient but also helps to induce relaxation. This herb is also said to help in lowering high blood pressure. While not many people use this herb for cooking purposes, its flowers can be used in baking while leaves can be used in the same way rosemary is used.

Such herbs can be grown in your back yard so that you can access them with ease and also be sure that what you are using as a remedy for one complication will not bring on other complications. This is because when you grow something in your backyard, you have the opportunity to grow it organically – without using chemicals. This will help you to avoid other diseases that come as a result of consuming foods that have been sprayed with herbicides and pesticides, which are usually loaded with harmful chemicals.

Chapter 4: How to Lower Your Blood Pressure with Exercise

There is nothing bad about getting more exercise, whether you have high blood pressure or not. Research has shown, beyond doubt, that exercise has a positive effect on lowering blood pressure significantly and also prevents hypertension from occurring in the first place. Researchers from IQWiG – Institute for Quality and Efficiency in Health Care, Germany – and from the Graz University Hospital in Austria, looked at the result from a number of studies.

They found eight studies, with a total of 800 people suffering from hypertension, which focused on whether exercise would help to lower their blood pressure. Each person was monitored for a period of up to 12 months although most studies lasted for an average of 6 months. Four of the studies concentrated on regular consultations, each recommending more activity and whether the person took the advice or not. The other four studies consisted of people who were given a training program to do. The activities in the program were jogging, fast walking, cycling and aerobics and each session lasted for 30-60 minutes on between three and seven days per week. The result showed that getting more exercise lowered the systolic value by between 5 and 8 mm HG.

Before you start any kind of exercise program to lower your blood pressure you should speak with your doctor first. They may be able to suggest certain types of exercises that you should do and definitely should not be doing and will monitor your progress.

When do you need your doctor's permission before indulging in an exercise regimen?

It is always great to seek your doctor's advice before starting any exercise routine more so if:

- You are obese or over weight

- You smoke

- You have a family history of heart related complications that occur before 55 years

- You are a man who is older than 40 years or a woman above 50 years

- You have previously suffered a heart attack

- You are not sure if your health is great

- You have a chronic health complication, for example high cholesterol levels, high blood pressure

- You feel pain in your chest or experience dizziness with exertion

- If you are on any kind of medication. This is because some medications do not support rigorous exercises

Exercise doesn't mean you have to join an expensive gym either. Any kind of exercise works as long as you are moving around and your heart is beating faster than it would normally or you are breathing harder. Go for a brisk walk, go swimming, and do some gardening, anything that gets you moving.

What is the Best Type of Exercise?

There are three main types of exercise that you should be doing to help lower your blood pressure:

- **Aerobic, or cardiovascular** – helps to lower blood pressure and strengthen the heart muscle. Includes activities like jump rope, walking, cycling (outdoor or stationary) jogging, skating, cross-country skiing, aerobics, water aerobics and swimming. You could also do house hold chores such as raking leaves, mowing the lawn or scrubbing floors, climbing the stairs. This is because any exercise that increases your breathing and heart beat rate is an aerobic exercise.

- **Strength training** – helps to build up stronger muscles that will assist you in burning off more calories. It is also very good for strengthening bones and joints.

- **Weight training** – This exercise will cause an increase in blood pressure temporarily during the exercise. This increase may be dramatic and it all depends on the amount of weight lifted. However, indulging in weight lifting has got long term effects on one's blood pressure, which outweigh the risk of a short-term spike.

If you want to indulge in weight lifting, yet have high blood pressure, you have to remember:

a) Never hold your breath during exertion for this will lead to a dangerous spike in your blood pressure. Just breathe continuously and easily with every lift.

b) Being a go-getter is great however it should be one step at time. For starters, going for lighter weights will help you, as you will not get strained a lot. The more you strain yourself, the higher your blood pressure gets. You could simply challenge your muscles by carrying lighter weights over and over again; you can increase the number of times you repeat the lifts as time goes by.

c) When lifting those weights, learn how to use proper form to reduce injury occurrences

d) When you start feeling dizzy or feel really out of breathe, it will be great for you to stop exercising. If you also feel any chest pain or pressure, put those weights down. Make it a habit to listen to your body.

However, you need to ask your doctor if it is okay for you to indulge in weight training exercises

- **Stretching** – to help make you more flexible, to be more supple, to move better and prevent injury.

How Often and How Much Exercise Should You Do?

The difficulty with exercising is knowing how much to do to have a positive effect and how to know when to stop because overdoing it will do you more damage in the long run. People will tell you that you can never get too much exercise but you can and you can end up running your joints, tearing ligaments and causing damage to your muscles.

Choose moderate activity, something like a brisk walk, and go for around 30 minutes per day for at least 5 days a week. If you don't have the time, go jogging – 20 minutes jogging, three or four days of the week will give you the same benefits.

If you lead a sedentary lifestyle, you will need to build up to this gradually. Take your time, as long as you are getting some exercise every day, it doesn't matter if it takes a few weeks to get to that level.

The first thing you must do, with any form of exercise, is warm up. Take at least 5 to 10 minutes to warm up and choose exercises like marching on the spot, pumping your arms. Move on to heel digs and knee lifts to help stretch your muscles gently and finish up with shoulder rolls and knee bends.

Next, it's time to step things up a bit but don't overdo it. The general rule of thumb with exercising is, if you can h old a conversation with someone you're doing OK but if you can belt out a tune, you need to increase the intensity a little otherwise you are not getting as much out it as you should be.

The last thing to do is cool down properly. Never ever just suddenly stop exercising; your muscles need to be cooled off gradually. Towards the end of your program, start to slow down a little and keep slowing things down for a few minutes. This is important for anyone but especially with people with high blood pressure.

If you are worried about not being able to stick to an exercise routine, guide yourself by these three tips:

- Make it fun to do and you'll enjoy it a lot more. This will also make you want to do it more often.

- Schedule it into your routine on a daily basis. Plan your exercise – if you can't fit an actual routine into your day then make some changes elsewhere – walk to the train station instead of getting the bus; get off the train or bus a stop earlier; use the stairs at work or in the department store instead of the lift or the escalator.

- Find someone to exercise with, it will be far easier for you to stay motivated and you will enjoy it far more.

How Safe is Exercise?

In terms of blood pressure, exercising and getting active is one of the single best things you can do to lower it and keep it down. If you are concerned about what you can do and how much you can do, speak with your doctor. They can advise you if there are any limits you should abide by.

When you do exercise, pay close attention to your body, to how it feels. To start with, it will feel as if your body is protesting but that's only because it has to get used it. That's normal and, given time and regular exercise, your body will begin to react positively.

It is also normal to sweat and to breathe harder, for your heart to beat faster than normal. If you are not experiencing any of these then you are not working out hard enough and you are not getting any of the benefits of exercise. However, if you find yourself suffering with shortness of breath, or you feel like your heart is going to fly out of you, slow down or stop for a rest. If you experience any pains in the chest, you feel very weak or dizzy, get feelings of pressure or pain in your shoulder, jaw, neck or arm, stop immediately and, if the symptoms do not go, call for immediate emergency treatment.

Keep it safe

- When exercising, you need to start slowly as this helps to reduce the risk of injuries while you are at it.

- Always remember to warm up before you start exercising and also cool down once you are done

- Do not over do it, build the intensity of your exercises slowly.

- Seek medical help should you start experiencing any of the signs below while exercising;

  a) Dizziness or faintness

  b) Excessive fatigue

  c) Pain in an arm or jaw

  d) Severe shortness of breath

  e) Irregular heart beats

Monitor your progress

The best way if not the only way to detect high blood pressure is to keep constant track of your blood pressure. Your doctor could take your readings for you or you could do it at home. When you already have high blood pressure, monitoring it at home will help you know if your exercise regimen is aiding high blood pressure lowering. When choosing to monitor your blood pressure from home, make sure that the readings are very accurate and you check your blood pressure before exercising and about an hour after exercises.

Exercise is good, it can be fun and it will certainly benefit you in more than one way but the key is not to overdo it. Next, I want to talk about the effects of stress on your blood pressure.

Chapter 5: How to Lower Your Blood Pressure by Reducing Stress

Stress does not actually cause high blood pressure but reducing stress will improve your health, which will help to lower your blood pressure. Situations that are stressful can cause your blood pressure to spike but only temporarily. However, many people believe that a buildup of short-term blood pressure spikes, over a period of time can lead to permanent hypertension. At this stage, there is little evidence, either for or against that notion but we do know that stress, on its own, as a one off will not raise your blood pressure long term.

Any activity that reduces your blood pressure will also reduce your levels of stress and exercise is one of the best remedies for that. For people with high blood pressure, anything that can help to reduce stress and make you healthier is going to have a positive effect on your blood pressure.

When you are experiencing stress, your body produces a lot more hormones than it would normally, generally causing your heart to speed up and your blood vessels to constrict. This causes your blood pressure to rise. When your body calms down, and you leave the stressful situation, your heart rate slows down and your blood vessels open up again, thus lowering your blood pressure.

While there is no real proof that stress is linked to high blood pressure in the long term, there is proof that other activities that cause stress to your body are. When we talk about stress, we are not necessarily talking about a situation that you find yourself in, like a heated discussion at work, being asked to do much in too short a time, for example. Although these things will cause you stress, there are other things that you may not link to stress.

For example, smoking, eating too much or not sleeping well cause your body to suffer stress and these can all cause high blood pressure. If you suffer from depression, anxiety or isolation, while these on their own do not cause stress, they can cause heart disease, which, in turn, will cause your blood pressure to go up.

A rise in your blood pressure, related to stress, can happen quickly but it can also drop just as quickly when the event or thing that has caused the stress disappears. However, while it is spiking rapidly, it could be damaging blood vessels, your kidneys and your heart in a similar way to long-term hypertension. Add to that your reaction to the stress – smoking, drinking or eating badly, perhaps – and your risk of high blood pressure increases even more, as well as your risk of stroke or heart attack.

So, how do we deal with this? While an instant reduction in stress may not lower your blood pressure long term, there are some strategies you can use to help you manage stress and make improvements to your health in other ways. Some of the things you can do are:

- **Make your schedule simpler** - Take the time out to review your to-do lists or calendar and look for the things that take your time up but don't make you feel as though you have achieved anything. It is these things that are not that important that cause you to rush jobs that are important, leaving you feeling stressed out and highly strung. Get rid of them or schedule them for another day.

- **Learn how to breathe** - That may sound daft to you; after all, you have to breathe to be alive. But, you can learn deep-breathing techniques that will help you to slow your breath and deepen it and you will find that you will relax.

- **Exercise** - Physical activity is great for busting stress. Make sure, as we talked about earlier that you get some advice from your doctor before you begin an exercise regime, especially if your doctor has already diagnosed you with hypertension. Exercises knocks stress on the head as well as reducing your systolic blood pressure significantly.

- **Learn yoga or meditation** - Both of these work to strengthen up your body, your mind and help you learn to relax as well as bringing your blood pressure levels down and kicking stress out of the door.

- **Sleep well** - You may think that you are getting enough sleep – after all, you sleep for 8 hours every night. The key to sleep is good sleep. It's no good sleeping for that long if you are restless, or only sleeping lightly, disturbed by every noise. God sleep means sleeping deeply, without interruption, and giving your body a chance to rest. Plus, facing problems on a lack of decent sleep will only make them seem worse.

- **Change your perspective** - When you are facing problems and trying to deal with them, bite back your tendency to complain. Take the time out to acknowledge how you feel about the problem and then turn your focus to finding a solution that works.

- **Get to know what triggers stress in your life** — If you are to deal with stress, you need to get to the bottom of it. What is it that causes you to get stressed out? This may necessitate you to change some beliefs that you have had over the years, change how you look at some situations or even learn to look at things from the positive side and not the negative side only.

- Find what works effectively for you, keep your mind open and be willing to experiment. Be open to change, accept help where it is offered and start enjoying your new stress-free life.

Chapter 6: How to Lower Your Blood Pressure by Leading a Healthy Lifestyle

Most diseases in our lives are caused by the unhealthy lifestyles we choose to lead. When you live a healthy lifestyle, it means that you have made the right choice and health complications such as high blood pressure are not likely to hit you. When we choose to let go of vices such as smoking, eating foods high in fructose, daily consumption of coffee, excessive consumption of alcohol we are on our way to a healthy life. Here are some lifestyle changes you need to adopt:

- **Losing weight** - Are you obese or overweight? Then you need to consider losing that weight because it is one of the leading causes of high blood pressure.

- **Exercise regularly** - An active life is not susceptible to high blood pressure or any of the diseases related to an inactive life. Go to the gym, take brisk walks or join an aerobics class for that much needed active life. Do this a number of times every week.

- **Measure you BMI** - You may ask yourself if you really need to lose weight, if that is the case, ask your doctor to measure your BMI-Body Mass Index and waistline. These readings will tell you if you are prone to high blood pressure or not. A healthy waistline is 40 inches for men and 35 inches for women.

- **Eat healthy** - What are you feeding your body with? If your blood pressure is high as well as your weight, you need to remove all sugars and grains from your diet more so fructose until your blood pressure and weight have got to a normal level. When one consumes bread (any type), potatoes, rice, or corn his or her insulin levels and blood pressure remain high.

When digested, fructose breaks down into a series of waste products that are not good for your body such as uric acid. Uric acid will divide your blood pressure by keeping nitric acid from your blood vessels with. Nitric acid helps vessels to maintain elasticity, therefore, when it is suppressed it increases high blood pressure. Increased uric acid levels in one's body cause hypertension.

You also need to do away with processed and fast foods and indulge more in fruits, vegetables and low fat diary products. Look out for DASH diets.

- **Reduce the amount of sodium you consume** - By taking a lot of salt in your diet; you are consuming a lot of sodium, which is not healthy for you. Choose to stop passing the saltshaker.

- **Stop smoking** - It is addictive therefore the habit is not easy to break; however, it is not impossible. Talk to your doctor for help on how to stop smoking because it is not doing your blood pressure any good.

- **Limit the amount of alcohol you consume** - You love meeting with your friends and you drink until the crate is empty. It is fun but not for long because your body's blood pressure is getting affected in the long run. Men, reduce it to 2 drinks a day and women, 1 in a day.

- **Increase your levels of vitamin D** - People that live further from the equator are more susceptible to high blood pressure because sun exposure is limited. Exposure to sunshine has dramatic effects on one's blood pressure like,

    a) Lack of vitamin D is also associated with insulin resistance and metabolic syndrome, obesity, elevated cholesterol levels, high blood pressure.

    b) When your body is exposed to the sun, vitamin D is produced. However, limited vitamin D causes an increase in the production of parathyroid hormone which increases your blood pressure

    c) Vitamin D also negatively inhibits renin-angiotensin system in your body, which helps in regulating blood pressure. Insufficient vitamin D will trigger inappropriate renin-angiotensin system (RAS) activation hence hypertension.

    d) Getting exposed to UV rays is also said to lead to the release of endorphins, which are chemicals in the brain responsible for producing pain relief and euphoria feelings. Naturally, endorphins help with stress relieving, stress management and most importantly deal with hypertension.

- **Reduce on that stress** - Chronic stress leads to hypertension, however, even occasional stress can lead to hypertension if the person resorts to unhealthy eating, smoking or drinking alcohol while in that state. Take time and reflect on your life to find out what causes stress in your life and try to avoid those situations. This may take sometime but it is worth it for your health. You may also have to change your belief system because it may be causing you to get stressed. Change how you live your life to live longer.

- **Do regular blood pressure checks at home and see your doctor regularly** - Doing blood pressure checks regularly even at home will greatly help you keep tabs on your blood pressure. You need to alert your doctor should any complications arise. In addition to that, visiting your doctor as regularly as the need is will go a long way in avoiding any bad health occurrences

Chapter 7: High Blood Pressure During Pregnancy and How to Deal With It Naturally

It is not mandatory that every woman will have high blood pressure during pregnancy; however, due to changes happening in the body, some women get it. Sometimes, someone will have high blood pressure before pregnancy while other times it will only show up during pregnancy. However, whatever the case, it needs to be dealt with so fast.

Here are some high blood pressure types that happen during pregnancy:

- Chronic hypertension - This is high blood pressure that was present before conception or that appears when the woman is 20 weeks pregnant. However, because high blood pressure barely has symptoms, it may not be easy to determine its presence.

- Gestational hypertension - Women with this kind of hypertension develop high blood pressure after 20 weeks of pregnancy. With this kind of hypertension, no protein is found in the urine and there is no sign of damage to the organs. For some of the women with this kind of hypertension, the condition transcends into preeclampsia.

- Chronic hypertension coupled with superimposed preeclampsia - Some women who have high blood pressure before conception develop more detrimental high blood pressure coupled with protein in their urine and/or other health problems during pregnancy.

- Preeclampsia - There are times when gestational or chronic hypertension leads to preeclampsia. Preeclampsia is a complication during pregnancy that is characterized with signs of organ damage and high blood pressure. It usually occurs after 20 weeks of pregnancy. If left untreated, preeclampsia could lead to serious or fatal complications for baby and mother. Earlier on, preeclampsia was only diagnosed when a pregnant woman with high blood pressure had protein in her urine. However, experts now say that a pregnant woman can have eclampsia with no protein in her urine.

Effects of high blood pressure during pregnancy

- Placental abruption - When a woman has preeclampsia, chances are high that placenta abruption will occur. Placenta abruption is when the placenta separates from the uterus' inner wall before birth. Severe bleeding and damage to the placenta will occur should severe abruption happen. This is life threatening for the baby and mother.

- Reduced blood flow to placenta - When there is a reduction in the amount of blood getting to the placenta, the fetus is likely to receive fewer nutrients and less oxygen. This will lead to a preterm baby, slow baby growth and low birth weight for the baby. Premature babies are likely to have problems with breathing.

- Premature delivery - There are times when the baby has to be born early in order to prevent life threatening complication from happening to the mother, baby or both.

- Cardiovascular diseases in the future - When one has preeclampsia, the chances of getting heart related diseases are high. The risk gets even higher when a mother has battled with preeclampsia more than once or has had a preterm birth. To minimize this risk, the mother has to maintain a healthy weight, consume lots of vegetables and fruits, quite smoking and exercise frequently before and after delivery.

More information on preeclampsia

There are times when preeclampsia develops without symptoms. In some instances, the high blood pressure will develop gradually while other times it will have a sudden occurrence. Therefore, monitoring your blood pressure is very important for blood pressure increment is preeclampsia's first sign. If a blood pressure reading that is 140/90 or more is recorded twice within 4 hours, it is abnormal.

Other symptoms of preeclampsia include:

- Severe headaches

- Nausea or vomiting

- Upper abdominal pain mostly under the ribs on the right

- Excess protein in the urine

- Kidney problems

- Vision problems such as blurred vision, temporary vision loss, light sensitivity

- Reduced urine output

- Impaired liver functionality

- Reduced levels of platelets

- Short breathes due to fluid in the lungs

Sudden gain in weight, and edema more so in the hands and face occur when one has preeclampsia, however, these things also occur in a normal pregnancy. Therefore they are not conclusive signs of preeclampsia.

Treatment of high blood pressure during pregnancy

Medicines during pregnancy affect the baby but there are some medicines meant to lower blood pressure that are safe for the mother and baby. However, medications like angiotensin receptor blockers (ARBs), angiotensin converting enzyme (ACE) inhibitors and rennin inhibitors should never be taken during pregnancy.

Treating high blood pressure is important least the mother risks getting a stroke, heart attack and many other high blood pressure related health issues that do not go away during pregnancy. High blood pressure is also greatly harmful to the unborn baby.

Before a pregnant woman can take any medication to keep the blood pressure in check, the help or advice of a medical practitioner will be very important. The medication should be taken as prescribed and at no time should the medication be stopped halfway or adjusted for that poses health threats.

How can the risks of this complication be reduced?

Every expectant mother needs to know that when she takes care of herself, she is also taking care of her baby or babies. For example,

- Eat healthy foods - Eat foods that are low in sodium, high in potassium and lots of vegetables and fruits.

- Go for your antenatal visits - Going to visit your medical practitioner regularly would help you in many ways such as preventing an impending complication.

- Stay active - Not all exercise regimens is accepted during pregnancy but consult with your doctor on what to do and what to avoid.

- Take your medicines as prescribed - Your doctor will give you the appropriate medicine to keep your blood pressure in check, all you need to do is take it as prescribed.

- Know what and what not to do - Let go of the cigarettes, alcohol, illegal drugs and the like. Avoid taking over the counted medicines.

Research continues to be made regarding ways to prevent preeclampsia however nothing conclusive has come through.

Natural remedies for high blood pressure during pregnancy

Many women think that they share a circulatory system with their unborn babies, however, that is not true because the unborn baby's circulatory system has no direct connection with that of the mother. The fetal heart and not that of the mother pumps its blood through its own arteries and veins. In addition to that, the placenta is the fetus' respiratory system because the baby's lungs are not functional during pregnancy. The mother's blood is filtered through the placenta and it goes to the umbilical cord before getting to the baby. At that time, it is safe and at a normal pressure. Normal fetal blood pressure is 30mmHg by 20 weeks, 45mmHg by 40 weeks. Therefore mothers need not worry that because they have got blood pressure so will their babies. Nonetheless, when a mother takes care of herself it goes long way in saving the unborn baby from a series of health complications. Here are some natural remedies to high blood pressure during pregnancy:

- Take less salt - a study conducted in 1991 at the Medical College of St. Bartholomew Hospital by the Department of Environmental and Preventative medicine showed that reducing the amount of salt in one's diet helped in lowering blood pressure. There is a lot of salt in processed foods so you might want to avoid them.

- Consume plant proteins - Studies have shown that proteins from plants have the ability to lower high blood pressure. Plant proteins can be got from lentils, soy products, nuts and some other pulses.

- Potassium - The National Heart, Lung and Blood Institute vouches for potassium as a remedy to high blood pressure. The recommended daily intake is 4,700 mg. Sources of potassium are raisins, bananas, lima beans, potatoes and avocados.

- Magnesium - The Good Hope Hospital's Department of Obstetrics and Gynecology in the UK notes that magnesium sulphate is great for pregnant women who stand a risk of eclampsia. Magnesium is also great for women who have got high blood pressure that has been brought on by preeclampsia or pregnancy.

- Calcium - Portland's Oregon Health Sciences University's Division of Nephrology and Hypertension carried out a study that revealed that a 1000 mg supplement of calcium can help in lowering high blood pressure.

- Keep a healthy weight - Even when you are pregnant, it is important to ensure that your weight is not leading to obesity. It is important for a woman to get to know what her BMI is before pregnancy so that she can keep tabs on her weight as the pregnancy advances. If your BMI were normal, a weight gain of 25 to 30 pounds would be okay. However, if you were underweight before getting pregnant, then a weight gain of 28 to 40 pounds will be great. An obese woman is advised not to exceed 20 pounds of weight gain during pregnancy. Most weight is gained during the 3rd trimester so every woman needs to make sure that the 1st and 2nd trimesters do not see her shoot in weight. With a reasonable weight, high blood pressure will be kept at bay.

- Exercise - Tulane University, New Orleans in 2002 carried out a study that showed that indulging in aerobics goes a long way in affecting your blood pressure positively. Pregnant women cannot indulge in all exercises; however, gentle exercises would be great. Consulting with a medical practitioner about which exercises to indulge in would be great.

- Rest - When anyone more so a pregnant woman has high blood pressure, resting will help lower it. Depending on its severity, she might be hospitalized or told to rest at home. Laying down and taking that weight off your feet, receiving fewer visitors will greatly help to lower high blood pressure.

- Avoid smoking - Many research works have shown that smoking before, during and after pregnancy is not good at all. This is because smoking greatly increases preeclampsia hence posing a danger for the baby and mother.

- Avoid any form of stress - Stress will trigger much more than just a temporary spike in blood pressure but a future of hypertension. Stress needs to be avoided more so during pregnancy and if you can not do away with stress causing factors, then take up some de-stressing measures like consuming foods that help in stress reduction such as foods rich in Omega 3 and 6- Salmon fish.

- Massage - London South Bank University in 2007 carried out a study that revealed that a facial massage for a little as 20 minutes can help in lowering systolic blood pressure.

Hypertension during pregnancy is life threatening and it needs to be treated as fast as possible. However, a pregnant woman needs to make sure that she attends antenatal classes or endeavor to go for the scheduled doctor visits so that conditions such as these are taken care of before they get out of control.

Chapter 8: High Blood Pressure Among Children and How to Deal With It Naturally

While it is mainly common among adults, children also develop high blood pressure. It is easy to take a blood pressure reading among adults and tell that someone has high blood pressure but it is not the same among children. This is because their blood pressure changes as they grow. Most times, sufferers of high blood pressure have a similar blood pressure reading like that of the child next door though sometimes it is higher. High blood pressure among children depends on 3 things:

- Gender

- Age

- Height

High blood pressure in children below 10 years is mainly caused by underlying medical conditions. High blood pressure may also occur among babies and it usually comes about when the baby was a preterm or has problems with his or her kidneys or heart. However, children may develop high blood pressure for the same reasons adults do, such as lack of exercise, poor eating habits, obesity and the like.

Therefore it goes without saying that lifestyle changes like exercising, eating healthy foods can also help children to lower their blood pressure. However, for some children, medication may also be needed.

Hypertension among children does not show symptoms most times.

When to make that visit to the doctor

Since high blood pressure among children is mainly brought on by an underlying health complication, it is not really necessary to go and see a doctor simply to take a blood pressure reading for your child. However, during routine health checkups or doctor's appointments, parents need to ensure that they have the children's blood pressure checked. This should start at 3 years.

Is your child a preterm baby? Does he or she have congenital heart disease? Was his or her birth weight low? Does your child have kidney problems? If your answer is yes to any of those questions, then you need to start doing blood pressure checks right from infancy.

If for any reason you are concerned that you child may have a factor or element in them that makes them susceptible to high blood pressure, talk to the child's pediatrician. This doctor will tell you what to do, may be recommend more regular blood pressure checks.

Causes of hypertension among children

Just like earlier stated, high blood pressure among children is usually caused by underlying medical issues like hormonal disorders, heart problems, genetic conditions or kidney diseases.

In older children, more so those that are overweight, the real cause is usually unknown.

High blood pressure among children may also be caused by some medications. However, once it is discovered and these medications are stopped, the blood pressure returns to normal.

However, there are also those who get high blood pressure because of the unhealthy lifestyles they lead.

Essential or primary hypertension

This is a kind of high blood pressure that comes into being without any underlying condition causing it. It is often among older children and adolescents. There are risks that lead to one developing this type of high blood pressure and they include:

- High cholesterol and triglycerides

- Family history of high blood pressure

- A high fasting blood sugar level or type 2 diabetes

- Obesity or being over weight (a BMI that is over 25)

Secondary hypertension

This is a type of high blood pressure that is caused by an underlying health condition. It is usually among young children. Other health issues that could cause this type of hypertension are:

- Hyperthyroidism

- Adrenal disorders

- Chronic kidney disease

- Pheochromocytoma which is a rare tumor in the adrenal gland

- Conditions affecting the kidneys, such as lupus

- Heart problems, such as coarctation of the aorta

- Renal artery stenosis which is where the artery to the kidney narrows

- Polycystic kidney disease

Complications

When a child gets high blood pressure and it is not taken care of immediately, then this child is most likely to have it even as an adult.

The most common complication that children with high blood pressure have is sleep apnea. This is a condition where a child snores or experiences abnormal breathing when sleeping.

Parents need to pay close attention to any breathing problems that their children may have when asleep because most children with breathing problems while sleeping like sleep apnea usually have high blood pressure. This is more so in children with weight problems.

When a child's blood pressure problems transcend into adulthood, this child is at risk of:

- Heart failure

- Heart attack

- Kidney failure

- Stroke

Preparing for a visit to the doctor

Most times, your child's blood pressure will be checked during routine checks. However, if you have noticed that your child may be at risk of developing high blood pressure, you need to see a doctor before matters get out of hand. When going to see a doctor about your child, you need to prepare for it since these visits are usually brief. Here are some things you can do so that you get to cover enough ground during the visit:

- Note any signs and symptoms – Even though high blood pressure rarely has symptoms, there may be some other signs or symptoms you may have noticed over time that the doctor needs to know about such as childhood illness.

- Write down important personal information – this will include family history of high blood pressure, stroke, heart disease, and diabetes. You can also write down any recent life changes you child has undergone or any major stresses the child may face if any.

- Write down all the medications – write down all the medicines your child has been taking, supplements and vitamins inclusive

- Go with a relation or family – If it is possible, go with someone for comfort, company and to remind you of anything you might have forgotten from what the doctor said. It is not easy to soak up all that the doctor says to you because you could be too emotional to get it all.

- Prepare to discuss your child's diet – Seeing that high blood pressure is brought on by a number of things such as what we eat, you need to discuss with the doctor what your child may eat and what not to eat. You could also be referred to dietician who will help you and guide you on how to prepare foods without necessarily dropping those favorite meals or losing flavor.

- Prepare to talk about exercises- An active body is needed if we are to beat high blood pressure, therefore you need to talk to the doctor about exercises for your child and which one's would be the best to indulge in.

- Write down any questions you may have for the doctor – this is mainly because writing them down helps you to exhaust them within the short time you are with the doctor. You could ask questions such as:

    a) What foods should my child avoid or eat?

    b) Is there need for medication?

    c) What level of exercise is appropriate?

    d) What tests will my child have to take?

    e) How often must I see a doctor to check my child's blood pressure?

f) Is it okay to monitor his or her pressure from home?

g) How do I do it?

h) Are there any alternative approaches to what you have suggested?

i) Is there a need to schedule an appointment with a specialist?

j) Can I try some generic alternatives to treat my child's high blood pressure?

k) Is there anywhere I can get some more information on this?

In addition to the questions you prepare, do not feel shy to ask any questions should you fail to understand something during the visit.

You also need to know that the doctor will ask you some questions that are key to finding the best way to treat your child. These questions will include:

- Is there any one in your family that has high blood pressure, high cholesterol or heart disease?

- When was the last time your child had a blood pressure check? What was the reading?

- What does your child feed on?

- Does your child indulge in physical activities or exercises?

Tests and diagnosis

Testing for high blood pressure is painless since no prick is done but an inflatable arm cuff and a pressure measuring gauge. The size of the cuff will vary with the circumference of the child's arm and a tight squeeze will be felt as the cuff is inflated. In addition to no pain, you do not have to wait for your results, as you will be told as soon as the test is done.

High blood pressure readings have 2 numbers; the systolic pressure, which is the 1st or upper one, then the diastolic reading which is the 2nd or bottom reading. Systolic pressure is that pressure in your child's artery at every heartbeat while diastolic pressure is the blood pressure between heartbeats.

Blood pressure varies among children therefore what may seem high for a 5 year old boy may be normal for a 10 year old girl. The sex, age and height of the child determine if the blood pressure reading is normal. The doctor will tell you if your child's pressure is normal or not.

You need to know that one blood pressure test is not enough to determine whether your child has got high blood pressure or not. Usually, a doctor will ask you to go for up to 3 tests before he or she can give you any conclusive diagnosis.

Once the doctor has told you that your child's high blood pressure is not normal, then you need to ensure that it is checked every 6 months after the diagnosis.

Your child could be diagnosed with pre-hypertension or hypertension. If this is the case, the doctor will ask you to take the child for some more tests to find out if there are any conditions causing the rise in blood pressure. These tests include:

- Urine sample test (urinalysis)

- Ultrasound of the child's kidneys

- Blood test to find out the functionality of the kidneys, to know the blood cell count and to check the blood sugar

- Echocardiogram – this is a test to check the blood flow through one's heart just in case the doctor suspects that a heart complication is the cause of the high blood pressure

However, there will be times when the doctor finds it difficult to diagnose high blood pressure or sees a need to monitor the child's treatment. In such instances, he or she will recommend ambulatory monitoring. This is where a child wears a device that will measure his or her blood pressure all day long. This practice is not so common and some more research is still being done regarding its efficiency in helping doctors diagnose and treat blood pressure among children. This device is mainly used for children who tend to be nervous during the doctor's visit. This is because such children may have white coat hypertension – temporal rise in blood pressure that is caused by anxiety at the sight of a doctor.

Treating high blood pressure among children

Despite the fact that sometimes the causes of high blood pressure among children are unknown, the ways on how to treat it do not differ much from how it is treated among adults. Nonetheless, scientists are trying to find a rather effective means to treat hypertension among children. One thing that parents need to do is to work closely with doctors in order to get a suitable work plan for the child. Here are a few general ways on how to deal with high blood pressure in children:

- Watch his or her weight – When a child is over weight or obese, the risk of developing high blood pressure is greatly increased. Exercising regularly, eating healthy foods can help in losing excess weight. Ask the pediatrician to help you in setting weight loss goals for your child. You may also be referred to other medical practitioners to help you set up a working weight loss plan.

- Medications should be taken – If your child has got severe high blood pressure or it is not responding to changes in lifestyle, some medicines may be given. The parents need to make sure that their children take these medicines as prescribed. There is still a difficulty in finding the right combination of medicines to deal with high blood pressure with very few side effects. However, the drugs that are being used now are:

- ACE inhibitors, calcium channel blockers, and alpha-blockers - which help to stop the blood vessels from getting tightened up.

- Diuretics – These help to lower the amount of fluid in the child's body which helps the body to get rid of excess sodium

- Beta-blockers – These medications prevent the body from producing the adrenaline hormone. Adrenaline is a stress hormone and it makes one's heartbeat harder and faster. It also causes the blood vessels to tighten. All these make the blood pressure to go up.

- Follow the DASH eating plan – Dietary Approaches to Stop Hypertension eating plans focus on consuming less fat and saturated fat while consuming more fresh vegetables and fruits and whole grain foods. They also ensure that the amount of salt consumed in reduced. The help of a dietician will come in handy to find ways on how goals will be met without letting go of favorite foods and flavor.

- Avoid smoking – Tobacco smoke is known to cause high blood pressure. It also directly damages the child's blood vessels and heart. It is the parent's obligation to protect this child from passive and active smoking. The children should also be educated about the dangers of smoking since they will not always be in the reach of parents or guardians.

How to Help a Child with High Blood Pressure

In as much as the above guidelines have been given, this child needs a lot more help to be able to keep the blood pressure down. The following steps can be taken:

- Make the issue of change in diet and exercises a family thing. Let everyone in the family take part in these changes so that the child will not feel alienated and the whole family gains from the healthy adjustments

- Ensure that the child's blood pressure is checked as often as needed or as advised by the doctor

- Reduce the number of hours that this child spends watching TV and playing video games.

When a parent works with a medical practitioner to come up with a comprehensive health plan for the child, your child will be helped greatly and you can be assured of many years of great health. In addition to that, parents need to be vigilant regarding their children and their health. This is because some of the things we ignore are the ones that turn out to be so disastrous. You also need to remember that usually high blood pressure shows no signs.

Chapter 9: Myths About High Blood Pressure

Just like any other disease, high blood pressure has got a number of misconceptions surrounding it. As you find out if you or your loved one has got high blood pressure, there are some myths you need to know. You will be better armed to deal with the condition then. Here are some of the common myths about high blood pressure:

High blood pressure is not a big deal – In the early stages of high blood pressure, you may not notice any signs and symptoms. However, as time goes by, this high blood pressure could lead you to your grave. On a normal day, your heart will beat normally and blood will get pushed through vessels all round your body. When blood is pushed by your heart beat, it will push against your blood vessel sides. Blood vessels are flexible and widen and constrict as needed for good blood flow. However, for a number of reasons, your blood will push so hard on the vessels and this will indeed bring about an increase in blood pressure.

High blood pressure will cause damage to your heart, blood vessels, kidneys and many other body organs. In the long run, you might experience health complications such as a stroke or heart disease, which are some of the world's leading killers.

As scary as it is, it is true that some one can have high blood pressure without knowing it. That is why some doctors call it a silent killer and will tell you that it is a big deal.

High blood pressure will occur only when you drink lots of coffee – Many people still doubt the link between caffeine consumption and high blood pressure. Some studies have gone ahead to show that even when one does not drink coffee regularly but consumes soft drinks, drinks coffee, tea, takes chocolate, takes pain killers, their blood pressure can still go up though on a temporary basis.

More so, the body seems to tolerate caffeine effects when it is consumed over a long period of time. However, when you are going to have your blood pressure checked, it will be wise to stay away from caffeine for a number of hours so that you can get that much needed perfect reading. You may also want to talk to your doctor before consuming things that have caffeine in them such as coffee for caffeine makes heart conditions such as arrhythmia worse.

Poor diet and an inactive life are what solely cause high blood pressure – There are a number of lifestyle and diet factors that will obviously increase one's risk of developing high blood pressure. These factors include lack of regular activity, obesity, consuming a lot of salt, or being over weight. However, there are other high blood pressure risk factors that no one has control over such as:

- Ethnicity – High blood pressure is prevalent among South Asians, Africans Inuit or Métis heritage.

- Age – most people who are 65 years and over have high blood pressure

- Family history of hypertension

So high blood pressure is caused by a combination of factors and some of which cannot be controlled. Therefore, if you are in that bracket of uncontrolled risk factors, it will be great to talk to your doctor about your blood pressure so that he can give you some much needed advice. This will help you avoid impending and avoidable health complications.

High blood pressure cannot be prevented – You may have a loved one who is at a high risk of developing high blood pressure or it may be you. You do not have to despair with the thought that there is no way out of this health complication. Even when there are many risk factors, you need not lose hope because there are some steps you can take to prevent high blood pressure if you do not yet have it or to lower it if you already have it. Here are some of them:

- Eat healthy – In as much as you should eat healthy foods, such as those low in fat, sugar and salt, you should remember to eat only the amount of food that the body needs.

- Reduce the amount of alcohol you consume

- Maintain a healthy weight – You can do this by the help of exercises and eating healthy.

- Watch the amount of salt you eat - Most of the sodium we consume is mainly in salt and there is a lot of it in processed foods. You could also desist from adding more salt as you eat.

- Life is full of stressful events, however, for the sake of your health, reduce the stress in your life. This is because a faster and harder heartbeat, which is a result of chemicals produced by your body when it is under stress will cause your blood vessels to get tight. This makes blood pressure to increase.

- Avoid passive and active tobacco smoking for tobacco smoke has been said to increase one's blood pressure.

- Regularly exercising for at least 30 minutes daily for 5 days in a week will help you relieve stress and control weight

You could also ask your doctor for any other suggestions on how to prevent high blood pressure.

All is well as long as one number is normal – When blood pressure readings are taken, there are two numbers, one on top of the other. These numbers are not understood by many. The top number is for systolic blood pressure and it shows the force with which your blood is going through your blood vessels at every heartbeat.

The number at the bottom is diastolic blood pressure and it shows the force with which blood flows through your vessels in between heartbeats, when your heart is at rest.

Systolic blood pressure reading

a) Normal systolic blood pressure is 119 and below

b) Pre-hypertension is when the reading is between 120 and 139

c) One has high blood pressure when the reading is 140 and more

d) For those who are over 60 years, a systolic reading of 160 and above shows the presence of high blood pressure.

Diastolic blood pressure reading

a) When diastolic reading is 79 and below, diastolic blood pressure is normal

b) A reading of 80 to 89 shows the presence of pre-hypertension

c) When the diastolic reading is 90 and above, then one has got hypertension

Most people mind most about systolic rate and less about diastolic rate. However medics say that the heart can deal with a high systolic rate better than a high diastolic rate.

One's high blood pressure will vary throughout the day depending on what he or she is doing. Blood pressure will also change with time; systolic blood pressure will increase with increase in age while diastolic blood pressure reduces with age.

If any of the blood pressure readings is always above normal, you need to see a medical practitioner straight away. You and your doctor will come up with a way to deal with the high blood pressure before damage is done.

One abnormal blood pressure reading means I have high blood pressure –One reading cannot be conclusive about one's blood pressure status. You can only be diagnosed with high blood pressure or hypertension after a number of blood pressure readings, say 3 readings. You may also be advised to stay away from caffeine or any physical activity hours before a blood pressure reading is taken to ensure an accurate reading. This is because physical exercises and caffeine increase one's heart, which will not give the right blood pressure reading.

High blood pressure treatment – Many people believe that when one is diagnosed with high blood pressure, he or she has got to let go of their favorite foods, take drugs that cause very disturbing side effects. It is true that it could take some time before a suitable treatment plan is got and this is because high blood pressure usually has a number of underlying causes. Many people do not have specific cause of high blood pressure.

With your cooperation, your doctor will help you come up with a combination of treatments that will help you control your blood pressure. Your work plan may include the following:

- Weight control - when one is over weight or obese, the risk of developing high blood pressure is high. Therefore following the DASH diet and exercising regularly will help in losing weight.

- No smoking - Tobacco smoke will cause your blood pressure to increase and it also affects your vessels and heart. Ask your doctor for ways on how to quit the habit.

- DASH eating plan - Eating less fat and saturated fat and more fresh vegetables and fruits plus whole grain foods is what DASH eating plan is all about. Reduced use of salt, limiting the amount of alcohol consumed will help in lowering your blood pressure. The help of a dietician will go a long way in helping you to deal with your high blood pressure.

- Reduce the amount of alcohol taken - Taking a lot of alcohol will lead to an increased blood pressure so cutting it back will be great.

- Medicine - You will be given some medication by your medical practitioner to control your blood pressure. You may need to take lots of tablets and your health care provider may keep switching medicines for you or changing your dosages until the right combination of medication is found with very minimal side effects. High blood pressure medications include:

  a) Beta-blockers - These are meant to stop your body from producing adrenaline. Adrenaline is a stress hormone that causes the heart to beat faster and harder causing the vessels to tighten hence increased blood pressure.

  b) Diuretics - these help in reducing the amount of fluids in one's body hence lowering the excess sodium.

c) Calcium blockers and ACE inhibitors – these do help to keep the blood vessels in their original shape; elastic and not tight

Treatments do not work – If a patient can cooperate with his or her doctor and they come up with a comprehensive work plan on how to keep the blood pressure in check, the plan will work just fine. To get the best out of a program, the following steps must be taken:

- Visit your doctor as often as needed or as told. Make sure that you bring your home readings so that the doctor can see how the plan is working.

- Make sure that you check your blood pressure as often as needed or as recommended by your medical practitioner.

- Inquire from your doctor or pharmacist about your medication and its related side effects. This will help you to know when to call on your doctor should a problem arise.

- Follow your plan religiously and talk to your doctor if you have any problem with any part of the plan. You may be referred to other medical practitioners such as a dietician for more help.

When you learn more about high blood pressure and its detrimental effects to your body, you are on your way to controlling the condition hence a long healthy life.

If my blood pressure level increased, I will obviously feel it – Doctors and several other people have called high blood pressure a silent killer because in most cases, no symptoms will be seen. However, there are some people that believe that when their heart rate is okay, so is their blood pressure. But the rate at which your hear beats is in no way connected to your blood pressure. The only conclusive way to know your blood pressure reading is by getting your blood pressure checked by your doctor or any other qualified medical practitioner. You could also take time to learn how to measure your blood pressure on your own so you can be able to take blood pressure readings in the comfort of your home.

Salt causes high blood pressure, avoid it – In the 1940s, a researcher from Duke University, Walter Kemper, M.D was famous for treating high blood pressure by telling his patients to stop using salt. Later on, it was proved that reducing the amount of salt one takes helps in reducing hypertension. Scientists have however gone on to say that once one has a normal blood pressure, there is no need to take salt out of their diet or restrict it. They however assert that if one has high blood pressure, reducing the amount of salt they consume will help them to keep it low. However, people who do not want to reduce the amount of salt they consume have been said to increase the amount of potassium they consume by eating more potassium rich foods. This is because potassium will balance out the sodium in the body. Some Dutch researchers actually say that one who takes less potassium is at more danger than one who takes in more sodium. Potassium can be got from fruits, legumes, and vegetables such as, white potatoes, broccoli, bananas, spinach and most types of beans.

Emily Hoskins

At the end of the day, when you know what you are dealing with, you will be more equipped to win the battle because you will not feel overwhelmed in any way

References

http://imsear.hellis.org/bitstream/123456789/135234/1/ijbb2009v46n6p503.pdf

http://www.ncbi.nlm.nih.gov/pmc/articles/PMC3210006/

http://www.researchgate.net/profile/Nicola_Robinson2/publication/224903412_Cinnamon_in_glycaemic_control_Systematic_review_and_meta_analysis/links/0fcfd50adfa406cb3d000000.pdf

http://www.ncbi.nlm.nih.gov/pmc/articles/PMC3210006/

http://www.ncbi.nlm.nih.gov/pmc/articles/PMC3210006/

Conclusion

The dramatic rise in the number of people who suffer from high blood pressure is concerning and there is a need for all of us to take action to prevent and treat the condition. Keeping your blood pressure down minimizes your risks of heart disease, cardiovascular disease and strokes, not to mention diabetes.

While there are pharmacological solutions that may be necessary in some cases, the best way to prevent and treat hypertension is to make some lifestyle changes. Exercise has always been one of the best ways to lower blood pressure, both systolic and diastolic values. Add to that a healthy diet and a life that is free of stress and you are on the right road to lowering your blood pressure and to preventing it from rising above dangerous levels again.

We all have the right to a healthy life but we must take the steps needed to keep it healthy and prevention of disease and conditions like high blood pressure are down to us to control. I hope that this book has been helpful to you, that I have been able to give you some ideas on how to make the right changes to your life to combat hypertension.

Preview of My Other Books

If you are interested in improving your health then you may also be interested in some of my other Amazon Top Ranking books.

Here's a list of a few that you may be interested in checking out.

>>>Download today by following the below link<<<

Belly Fat: *The Healthy Eating Guide to Lose That Stubborn Belly Fat - No Exercise Required*

http://www.amazon.com/Belly-Fat-Stubborn-Exercise-Required-ebook/dp/B00SUDGRTW

Belly Fat: ***The Fast Metabolism Diet*** *- Speed Up Your Metabolism for Fast Weight Loss, Fat Loss and Body Transformation*

http://www.amazon.com/Belly-Fat-Metabolism-Weight-Transformation-ebook/dp/B00XRCZGXE

Gluten-Free: *The Healthy Lifestyle Guide to Gluten-Free Diets*

http://www.amazon.com/Gluten-Free-Healthy-Lifestyle-Cooking-Cookbook-ebook/dp/B00QPD88EG

Sugar Free: *9 Life Changing Reasons To Follow A Sugar Free Diet: The Healthy Lifestyle Guide To Sugar Free Diets.*

http://www.amazon.com/Sugar-Free-Changing-Lifestyle-Diabetes-ebook/dp/B00S4SUP6E

Vegan Diet for Beginners - *20 Easy & Delicious Vegan Recipes for Healthy Living*

http://www.amazon.com/Vegan-Beginners-Delicious-Vegetarian-Cookbook-ebook/dp/B00T3DQQZS

Smoothies: *14 Nutrient-Packed Smoothies to Help You Detox, Lose Weight and Feel Fantastic*

http://www.amazon.com/Smoothies-Nutrient-Packed-Weight-Fantastic-Smoothie-ebook/dp/B00TW9KBNG

Paleo Diet for Beginners: *Quick And Easy Paleo Recipes To Help You Lose Weight Fast - Easy And Delicious*

http://www.amazon.com/Paleo-Beginners-Recipes-Delicious-Lifestyle-ebook/dp/B00TUC75RU

Or for some awesome insights on how to live a more confident, relaxed life then check out these:

Self-Esteem For Women: *The Ultimate Women's Guide to Loving Yourself and Building High Self-Esteem*

http://www.amazon.com/Self-Esteem-Ultimate-Self-Esteem-confidence-ebook/dp/B00SQ6K316

Meditation For Beginners - *Deep Relaxation Techniques For Long Lasting Peace and Happiness*

http://www.amazon.com/Meditation-Beginners-Relaxation-Techniques-Mindfulness-ebook/dp/B00T6PMSOQ

www.ingramcontent.com/pod-product-compliance
Lightning Source LLC
Chambersburg PA
CBHW072250310526
45795CB00011B/622